Dr SEBI's Approved Food and Recipes for Regaining Total Health

Brian Q. Pellign

Copyright © 2020 by Brian Q. Pellign

All rights reserved. No part of this publication may be reproduced, distributed, or transmitted in any form or by any means, including photocopying, recording, or other electronic or mechanical methods, without the prior written permission of the publisher, except in the case of brief quotations embodied in critical reviews and certain other non-commercial uses permitted by copyright law.

ISBN: 978-1-63750-195-5

Dedication

This book is dedicated to late Dr. Alfredo Darrington Bowman, popularly known as Dr Sebi.

Table of Contents

DR SEBI'S APPROVED FOOD AND RECIPES FOR REGAINING TOTAL HEALTH 1

DEDICATION 3

INTRODUCTION 5

CHAPTER 1 9

   DR. SEBI DIET HEALING ALKALINE DIET 9
      Dr Sebi Diet Overview 11
      How To Begin With Alkaline Living 12
      Nutritional Guide Food List 13
      Great Things About The Dr. Sebi Diet 17
      Tips For Sticking with the Diet 21
      Why Follow the Dr Sebi Diet? 25
      Nutritional Guide and Food List 27

CHAPTER 2 31

   DR SEBI'S APPROVED HEALTHY COOKBOOK 31
      ORGANIC FOODS 31
      RAW VS. COOKED 31
      EATING PROPERLY 32

CHAPTER 3 71

   DR SEBI FOOD LIST 71
      Dr Sebi Food List - Recommended Nutritional Guide 73

CHAPTER 4 80

   DR SEBI RECIPES 80
      BREAKFAST 81
      LUNCH 85
      DINNER 89

Introduction

Do you want to learn more on foods, herbs, juice and smoothie recipes necessary to cure diabetes, high blood pressure and detox your organs through Dr. Sebi alkaline diet?

Its no secret that eating healthy can boost your brain and body.

Dr. Sebi diet originates from native Honduran, Dr. Sebi (real name Alfredo Darrington Bowman), who is acknowledged as a natural healer, herbalist, and intracellular therapist. The methodology of Dr. Sebi is quite interesting and involves focusing on natural, alkaline, plant-based foods and herbs while steering clear of acidic and hybrid foods that may damage the cell. By following a strategy of Alfredo Bowman (aka Dr. Sebi), you can prevent mucus build-up, which can result in the introduction of diseases.

Sticking with the Dr. Sebi long-term diet isn't that hard when you can see through the first couple of days.

The starting days could be challenging though as you will yet crave sugar.

It doesn't help that there exist numerous fast food choices everywhere and that a lot of restaurants don't have menu items that fit this lifestyle.

Dr. Sebi was a Honduran man with a very humble beginning and was known and addressed as an herbalist, pathologist or a naturalist in different regions of the world; he left the biosphere in 2016, his self-invented and established effective traditional therapy for diabetes, hypertension and organ cleansing is still helping millions of people with these conditions around the world.

For optimal health, it is vital that people eat only non-hybridized organically grown food product. Conventional or commercial produce is grown with pesticides, herbicides, synthetic fertilizers, and other chemicals that are toxic and bad for your body.

He created great strides in the world of natural health and wellness with the creation of his specialized diet. *Dr. Sebi said that there were six fundamental food groups: live, raw, dead, hybrid, genetically modified, and drugs, but his diet basically cut out all the food groups except live and raw food, thereby encouraging dieters to eat as closely to a raw vegan diet as possible.* These foods include foods like naturally grown fruits and vegetables, along with whole grains. *He has the believed that raw and live foods were "electric," which fought the acidic food waste in the body. So, with his approach to eating, Dr. Sebi established a list of foods that he deliberated to be the best for his diet.*

This book is written so as to give you all of the information you need to eat right and the type of fruits, food, herbs, juice and smoothie recipes, etc to eat to live healthy.

Chapter 1

Dr. Sebi Diet Healing Alkaline Diet

The motivation behind the Dr. Sebi diet originates from native Honduran, Dr. Sebi (real name Alfredo Darrington Bowman), who is acknowledged as a natural healer, herbalist, and intracellular therapist.

The methodology of Dr. Sebi is quite interesting and involves focusing on natural, alkaline, plant-based foods and herbs while steering clear of acidic and hybrid foods that may damage the cell. By following a strategy of Alfredo Bowman (aka Dr. Sebi), you can prevent mucus build-up, which can result in the introduction of diseases.

Dr. Sebi is the known founder of the USHA Healing Village located in Honduras, which not only provides healing, but also teaches people how exactly to live an alkaline life-style.

Doctors often assume that the Dr. Sebi herbs method of curing disease is ineffective because they were taught to trust in the medicine method of treating patients. This way of thinking resulted in Dr Sebi and his astounding herbal compounds appearing on front page news to be delivered to the Supreme Court in NY, accusing Dr Sebi of earning false claims of healing people and practicing medicine with no license.

However, many folks have stated that the Dr Sebi diet boosts has improved their health much better with the compounds from Dr Sebi which the herbal method of human healing spent some time working much better than the pharmaceutical method of medicine. Dr. Sebi's thoughts about nutritional compounds and herbal therapy are all popular throughout YouTube, assisting to teach and promote healthy living even after his demise.

Bowman has been an inspiration to numerous and is fairly a herbalist because he invented a method to heal deadly diseases which have been considered incurable. He was an herbalist for 40 years plus, and claims to heal folks from AIDS, asthma, cancer, diabetes, eczema, epilepsy, fibroids, cardiovascular disease, high blood circulation pressure, inflammation, Lupus, multiple sclerosis, and sickle cell among other health issues.

Dr Sebi Diet Overview

The Dr. Sebi Diet is absolutely a vegan, plant-based diet that restricts man-made food and hybrids.

The Dr. Sebi diet is about minimizing acidity in your foods and mucus within your body.

Dr. Sebi (also called Alfredo Bowman) believes that whenever you do both of these things, you create an alkaline environment within your body that makes it tough for diseases to survive in.

How To Begin With Alkaline Living

The mucus reducing alkaline diet from your preferred Dr. Sebi involves consuming from a proprietary nutritional guide and food list that are founded on 40+ several years of research identifying non-hybrid, alkaline foods while also indulging in essence herbal of cell food.

Naturally, many people lose weight when eating based on the Dr. Sebi plant-based, alkaline diet because they're eliminating waste, meat, dairy, and processed food items off their diet.

Quite often people combine fasting and herbs with the Dr.

Sebi diet too to greatly help with cleansing, healing a cell or two, and/or overall well-being. In such cases, they usually seek advice from a health-care provider or healthcare professional.

Nutritional Guide Food List

Nutritional Guide

Sticking with the Dr. Sebi long-term diet isn't that hard when you can see through the first couple of days.

The starting days could be challenging though as you will yet crave sugar.

It doesn't help that there exist numerous fast food choices everywhere and that a lot of restaurants don't have menu items that fit this lifestyle.

As an end result, you will need to get accustomed to preparing a whole lot of meals yourself from home.

To greatly help with this, we created a recipe book as a product/program that provides you all the information you have to eat right, map out your meals, and also have fun, flavorful recipes that stick to the Dr. Sebi diet.

What Does The dietary Plan Consist of?

The Dr. Sebi diet is a vegan, plant-based diet and a distinct segment version of the alkaline diet (Source: National Institute of Health). While following a diet, many also ingest herbs to nourish the cell, help cleanse them and heal them of decades of horrible consumption of food.

Dr. Sebi considers alkaline foods to be "electric foods" for your cell that is live and raw foods that are for the "healing of the body." Generally, Dr. Sebi reduces food into six categories:

i. Live

ii. Raw

iii. Dead

iv. Hybrid

v. Genetically modified

vi. Drugs

Herbalist Sebi says that you ought to focus on #1 and #2 (live and raw), while steering clear of #3 - #6.

This involves avoiding seedless fruits and veggies, weather-resistant crops for example corn, and anything with added vitamins or nutrients which may be difficult for individuals due to the fact that there are so many hybrid and genetically modified (GMO) vegetables and fruit offered in food markets.

According to Dr. Sebi, foods that are recommended for individuals that are looking to live healthy consist of ripe non-starchyables, fruit, butter, raw nuts and grains. Leafy greens, quinoa, rye, and Kamut may also play a big role in the Dr. Sebi diet.

Acidic foods including meat, poultry, seafood, or products containing yeast, alcohol, sugar, iodized salt, or whatever is deep-fried bring adverse effect to the body.

Replacing acidic foods with alkaline options will heal you from the side effects that acid produces.

Pursuing largely raw diets can appear unappetizing to acidic humans, nevertheless, you slowly begin to get accustomed to a raw diet as you detoxify your cells of toxins, resulting in the cure of disease.

Great Things About The Dr. Sebi Diet

Minimizing acid in foods immensely help to decrease mucus in your body, which creates an alkaline environment that means it is very hard for disease to get created. Including herbs in your cleansing approach is better still.

Dr Sebi Diet Weight Loss

This part is self-explanatory. Weight loss will happen when following diet since the Dr. Sebi diet includes natural vegetables, fruits and veggies, grains, nuts, and legumes.

It eliminates waste, dairy, meat, and processed food, so naturally, you will eventually lose weight. The Dr. Sebi diet serves as a cleanse/detox and reaps several benefits alongside your body thanking you.

Strong Disease Fighting Capability

A weak disease fighting capability is the consequence of illnesses and diseases. Some declare that they have strengthened their disease fighting capability and also have been healed of particular ailments by adhering to Dr. Sebi's diet regularly and everybody knows that medicine will not cure these diseases.

Reduced Threat of Disease

Acidic foods rot the mucous membrane of the cells and inner walls of your body that leads to a compromised system which makes disease possible and a remedy impossible. Consequently, consuming alkaline foods can decrease the threat of disease and support the body in obtaining what it requires to feed the nice cells.

Lower Threat of Stroke and Hypertension

Based on the National Institute of Health (NIH), first line therapies for any stages of hypertension include exercise and weight loss. However, results in one small cross-sectional research suggest a plant-based diet is definitely more important intervention than medicine and standard medical practice.

In addition, Everyday Health has discussed the advantages of a plant-based diet compared to medicine, stating that a plant-based diet can decrease plaque in the arteries and lower the threat of diabetes, stroke and cardiovascular disease in medical research they have reviewed.

As we discussed, the Dr. Sebi alkaline electric diet is a distinct segment version of the plant-based vegan diet.

Energy

Diets heavy in meat, white sugar and dairy could be a threat to your own body and energy. Concentrating on plant-based living is definitely a better strategy and can improve the energy that you exhibit regularly.

Increased Focus

Pursuing Dr. Sebi's teachings will clear brain fog, get you focused and less bothered by stressful circumstances that arise.

Even though you aren't sick, utilizing a plant-based methodology can help you live an extended and healthy life.

Tips For Sticking with the Diet

Unlike any other diet you've tried, sticking to this one will need time! While it could be difficult at first, the body will slowly get accustomed to this new method of eating. You might start to feel even more energized as you remove all of the bad foods you might have consumed previously. Below are a few recommendations and guidelines to check out to make this the most enjoyable experience possible.

Drink A lot of Water

According to Bowman, people ought to be drinking at least a gallon of drinking water per day. That is essential to ensuring that alkaline diet work to the very best of its ability. Alfredo recommends natural spring water instead of drinking water softeners or drinking water from a reverse osmosis system.

Other health organizations and nutritional professionals recommend a gallon of drinking water per day too. Remember that drinking water removes waste from your body while assisting in the absorption of nutrients and cushioning joints and organs.

Get Emotionally and Mentally Prepared

It is very likely that you have formed some strong habits eating certain types of foods daily that could make it very difficult to break or change your daily diet. Your friends and relations could also turn into a hindrance when trying to adhere to the Dr. Sebi diet. Before you begin this plan of action, spend time considering why you wish to change your diet and the obstacles, both mental and psychological, that you'll face.

Don't Quit Snacks

Yes! it's true! While you don't need to quit snacks, you ought to take snacks the proper way. What this means is rather than reaching for a bag of poker chips, eat a bit of fruit or create snacks predicated on the recommended nutritional guide.

Review the Approved Foods

Do your very best never to stray from the set of approved foods as it could hinder your outcomes. Although it may appear too difficult initially to consume from the selected list, you'll soon see it's easier than thinking particularly if you are ready mentally.

Add Whole Foods To Your Daily Diet

Do your very best to substitute packaged/processed foods with whole foods to what you eat regularly. You would need to avoid packaged/processed foods because they're filled with additives, which may be very addictive especially because so many have enhanced sugar that triggers food craving.

Cooking is vital

You will start to find that it's essential to cook when using the Dr. Sebi diet. The guides offer alkaline food recipes to make this technique easier. His guides walk you step-by-step through each alkaline meal. Once you start preparing your own meals, you'll observe how you can require your preferred dishes and prepare them using approved ingredients.

Why Follow the Dr Sebi Diet?

There are always a ton of diets available, but the majority of them are centered on reducing your weight and in addition incorporate foods which may be acidic.

Alkaline living isn't a diet…it is a means of life.

Think about it as growth, emanating out of darkness and into the light to ensure long term health and fitness.

According to Sebi, the Dr. Sebi diet will minimize illness due to mucus build-up in your body and you will use his non-hybrid alkaline based meals to keep up a wholesome body.

His products might help with cleaning body waste from one's body.

As stated before, the adjustment period might take time but just make an effort to power through the first couple of days and you'll be fine.

Make an effort to eat as many raw foods as possible, but

if you're struggling, Alfredo Bowman states that cooked foods aren't entirely the end of the world.

Also, do not microwave your meal if possible.

It is greatly suggested to consult your physician before starting the program.

Nutritional Guide and Food List

You might be wondering what foods you can eat. Although it seems like your alternatives are limited, they aren't and the Dr. Sebi diet is easy and achievable.

The majority of the non-hybrid foods on the nutritional guide are the following.

Vegetables:

Amaranth Greens, Wild Arugula, Asparagus, Bell

Peppers, Mexican Squash or Chayote, Garbanzo Beans (chickpeas), Kale, Lettuce (aside from Iceberg), Mushrooms, Mexican Cactus or Nopales, Okra, Onions, Squash, Tomato (cherry and plum), Zucchini.

Fruits:

Apples, Bananas, Orange, Berries, Cantaloupe, Cherries, Figs, Grapes -seeded, Limes, Mango, Melons -seeded, Papayas, Plums, Peaches, Pears, Prickly Pear (Cactus Fruit), Prunes, Raisins -seeded, Tamarind.

Nut products and Seeds:

Brazil Nuts, Hemp Seed, Raw Sesame Seeds, Walnuts.

Oils:

Essential Olive Oil, Coconut Oil, Grapeseed Oil, Hempseed Oil, Avocado Oil.

Spices and Seasonings:

Basil, Cayenne, Cloves, Dill, Habanero, Onion Powder, Oregano, Pure Sea Salt, Sage, Thyme.

What not to Eat:

Meat, dairy (eggs, milk, etc), garlic, white sugar, man-made food.

As the Dr. Sebi diet is strict, you might find the first couple of days to be extremely challenging.

Lucky for you we have recipes made available to you, and additionally, there are a great deal of videos on YouTube that would also be of help. Just make a search for each of the food recipes.

Popular recipes include meatless meatballs, alkaline based noodle recipe, and fluffy gluten-free waffles.

Chapter 2

Dr Sebi's Approved Healthy Cookbook

ORGANIC FOODS

For optimal health, it is vital that people eat only non-hybridized organically grown food product. Conventional or commercial produce is grown with pesticides, herbicides, synthetic fertilizers, and other chemicals that are toxic and bad for your body. Organic foods are grown without the utilization of the harmful substances; therefore they taste better, are nutritious and so are less dangerous to your bodies.

RAW VS. COOKED

During the greater part of our existence in this world, what choices did we've for food? What could we've eaten through the first 50,000 years before we found out fire, implements and tools to kill animals? The initial diet of Homo sapiens will need to have been fruits, vegetables, and nuts! How many other choices did we've? A raw, plant-based diet is the primary food staple throughout a large proportion of the annals of humankind! Before humans started out killing and eating dead animal carcass, berries, they ate fruits, leaves and nuts.

EATING PROPERLY

Are you dependent on food? Most of us have become dependent on certain foods. A lot of people have about 5 or 6 foods they are actually addicted to and have trouble releasing. These food types are usually hybrids which includes rice, beans, soy, breads, potatoes, potato chips, coffee, teas, sweets, chocolate candy, fish, carrot juice, which contains high content of sugar, most are also addicted to cigarettes.

Kamut Raisin Pancakes

- ✓ 2 cups of Kamut flour
- ✓ 1 cup of maple crystals
- ✓ 2 tsp of vanilla extract
- ✓ 1 2/3 tsp of seams powder
- ✓ 1/2 cup of almond milk
- ✓ 1/4 cup of raisins

Procedure:

i. Put Kamut flour, seamoss powder in a bowl

ii. Then add raisins, vanilla extract, and maple crystals

iii. Stir in almond milk

iv. Pour into heated pan and cook evenly on both sides.

Seamoss Breakfast Shake

- ✓ 4 bp of almond butter
- ✓ 1 cup of maple syrup
- ✓ 3 cups of almond milk
- ✓ 3 tsp of vanilla extract
- ✓ 2 tsp of cinnamon
- ✓ 1 tsp of seamoss
- ✓ 3-4 cups of water

Procedure:

i. In a blender, add warm water with seams then blend

ii. Combine almond butter, maple syrup, cinnamon, vanilla extract and almond milk

iii. Blend until smooth and serve.

Spelt Strawberry Waffles

- ✓ 2 cups of spelt flour
- ✓ 1/2 cup of almond milk
- ✓ 1/4 cup of water
- ✓ 1 tsp of seams
- ✓ 1/4 cup of agave nectar
- ✓ 1 tsp of vanilla extract
- ✓ 6 strawberries cut into small pieces.

Procedure:

i. Put spelt flour, seams, and strawberry pieces in a

clean bowl

ii. Add agave nectar, vanilla extract, normal water, and almond milk

iii. Mix together and pour into waffle maker and cook

Cream of Rye

- ✓ 1/2 cup of cream of rye
- ✓ 1/2 cup of water
- ✓ 1/2 cup of almond milk
- ✓ 1 tsp of vanilla extract
- ✓ 1/4 cup of agave nectar.

Procedure:

i. Pour water into a pot and boil

ii. Once boiling, have it opt from the fire

iii. Add cream of rye mix until thickens

iv. Add vanilla extract, agave nectar and milk

v. Stir then serve

Blueberry Spelt Muffins

- ✓ 1/4 tsp of sea salt
- ✓ 1/3 cup of maple syrup
- ✓ 1 tsp of baking powder 1/2 cup of sea moss
- ✓ 1/2 cup of sea moss
- ✓ 3/4 cup of spelt flour
- ✓ 3/4 cup of kamut flour
- ✓ 1 cup of almond milk
- ✓ 1 cup of blueberries

Procedure:

i. Preheat oven to 400F.

ii. Place baking cups in a muffin pan

iii. Combine flour, syrup, salt, baking powder, and seamoss together in a mixing bowl.

iv. Add almond milk then mix

v. Fold in blueberries

vi. Pour into baking cups and bake for 25-30 minutes

Spelt French Toast

- ✓ 2 slices of Spelt Bread

- ✓ 1 cup of Almond Milk

- ✓ 2 tsp of Quinoa flakes

- ✓ 2 tsp of spelt flour

- ✓ 2 tsp of maple crystals

- ✓ 1/2 tsp of sea salt.

Procedure:

i. Mix all ingredients together except the breads

ii. Dip bread into the mixture untill soak however not soggy.

iii. Add little olive oil to pan to lightly fry on both sides.

Kamut Puff Cereal

- ✓ 1/4 cup of agave nectar
- ✓ 1 cup of hot Almond milk
- ✓ 1/4 of raisins
- ✓ 1/4 cup of chopped almonds
- ✓ 1/4 cup of chopped dates

- ✓ 1 cup of kamut puffs

Procedure:

i. Mix almond milk with almonds, dates, agave nectar and cereal!

ii. Enjoy.

Papaya Breakfast Shake

- ✓ 2 cups of almond milk
- ✓ 1/2 cup of agave nectar
- ✓ 1 tsp of seams
- ✓ 1/2 cup of cool water
- ✓ 1/2 cup of fresh or frozen papaya.

Procedure:

i. Blend water and seamoss

ii. Add Papaya, milk, and agave nectar

iii. Blend till smooth and serve.

Cream of Kamut

- ✓ 4 cups of almond milk
- ✓ 2 cups of water
- ✓ 1/2 cup of kamut flour
- ✓ 1/2 tsp of vanilla extract
- ✓ 1 cup of maple crystals
- ✓ 1 tsp of cinnamon.

Procedure:

i. Make like cream of rye

Pasta Salad

- ✓ 2 boxes of spelt penne
- ✓ 2 avocados cut in small pieces
- ✓ 1/2 cup of sun dried tomatoes
- ✓ 1/2 cup of cut onions
- ✓ 1/4 cup of almond milk
- ✓ 1/4 cup of fresh lime juice
- ✓ 3 tbs of maple syrup
- ✓ 4 tbs of sea salt
- ✓ 3-4 dashes of cilantro
- ✓ 1/2 cup of essential olive oil

Procedure :

i. Cook the pasta as directed on package

ii. Add everything in a huge bowl

iii. toss until evenly distributed

Mushroom Patties

- ✓ 2 portabella mushrooms
- ✓ 1/2 cup bell peppers
- ✓ 1/4 tsp oregano 1 Pinch of cayenne pepper
- ✓ 1/4 couple of cilantro
- ✓ 4 tbs sea salt
- ✓ 1 tsp dill
- ✓ 2 tsp onion powder
- ✓ 1/4 cup of spelt flour

Procedure:

i. Soak mushrooms for 1 minute in spring water

ii. Remove and place in food processor with scallions and bell peppers

iii. Add cilantro, flour and all the other seasonings

iv. Mix thoroughly and make patties

v. Place them in heated pan with 2 tbs essential olive oil

vi. Fry on both sides until done (approximately three minutes each).

The Greatest Greens

3 bunches of mustard and turnips greens 1/2 of every

2 cups of chopped onions

1/4 cup essential olive oil

1 tsp of cayenne or chili powder

3 tbs sea salt.

Procedure:

    i.   heat pan then add onions, cook till golden brown

    ii.   add greens, cook down for 20 min.

    iii.   season with sea salt, and Cayenne or chili powder

Stuffed Bell Peppers

- 1/2 cup of quinoa
- 1 lb. oyster or brown button mushroom
- 2 green bell peppers
- 3 tbs olive oil
- 1/2 red bell peppers sliced fine
- 1/4 tsp of ground cumin
- 1/2 tsp nice basil

- ✓ 1/2 tsp dill

- ✓ 1/2 tsp sea salt

- ✓ 2 slices of kamut or spelt breads toasted, crumbled.

Procedure:

i. steam bell peppers until tender, then hollow out

ii. place quinoa grain in saucepan with water within the top

iii. cook over low heat until water is absorbed, then reserve

iv. sauté mushrooms and red bell peppers in essential olive oil

v. season inside bell peppers with some spices and essential olive oil

vi. mix quinoa, mushrooms, and red bell pepper with remaining seasonings

vii. stuff bell peppers with mixture, then sprinkle bread crumbs over the top

viii. bake in preheated oven at 250 degrees for 10-15 minutes

ix. serve hot and revel in with a green leafy salad.

Vegetable Mushroom Soup

- ✓ 1 lb oyster mushrooms, chopped
- ✓ 1 cup quinoa
- ✓ 1 small red and green bell pepper chopped
- ✓ 1 bunch spinach, washed, and steamed
- ✓ 2 tbs olive oil
- ✓ 1/2 lb kamut spiral pasta
- ✓ Spring water

- ✓ 2 onions chopped finely
- ✓ 2 large chayote squash, peeled and chopped
- ✓ 2-3 bunches kale
- ✓ 1 clove
- ✓ 1/2 to: marjoram, Rosemary, oregano, thyme, red pepper, and cumin.

Procedure:

i. put essential olive oil in hot skillet

ii. sauté mushrooms, bell peppers, and onions slowly for 20 minutes

iii. add mushroom mixture in a soup pot and fill with spring water

iv. add chayote squash

v. add thyme, marjoram, Rosemary, oregano, red pepper, cumin, clove and quinoa

vi. Simmer for 45 minutes

vii. add Kamut Pasta and simmer for 15 minutes

viii. add spinach, stir and serve when tender.

Vegetable Patties

- ✓ 1 bunch of broccoli cut fine

- ✓ 1 couple of kale greens cut fine

- ✓ 2 chayote squash diced

- ✓ 1/2 red and green peppers chopped

- ✓ 1 medium yellow onion chopped fine

- ✓ 1 pinch of African red pepper 3 tbs essential olive oil

- ✓ 1/4 cup seamoss powder

- ✓ Spring Water

✓ Kamut Flour

Procedure :

i. heat skillet with 3 tbs essential olive oil

ii. add onion, bell pepper, chayote squash, African red pepper and ground cumin, sauté 2-3 minutes

iii. add broccoli and kale simmer 10-12 minutes

Preparation for Kamut flour:

i. mix seamoss with enough flour and normal water to produce a dough

ii. roll on floured board and cut into 10cm diameter circles

iii. place cooked vegetables on half of the circle

iv. fold other half to cover the vegetables

v. use a fork to pinch the edges closed

vi. place patties on lightly greased baking sheet and

bake 20-30 minutes or until golden brown.

Homestyle Okra

- ✓ a1b fresh okra diced
- ✓ 2 soft tomatoes
- ✓ 1/2 yellow onion chopped fine
- ✓ 1/4 tsp ground cumin
- ✓ 4tbs olive oil
- ✓ 1/4 tsp African red pepper
- ✓ 1/4 tsp. sassafras
- ✓ 1/4 tsp. sea salt
- ✓ cooked wild rice or quinoa

Vegetable Stir Fry Medley

- ✓ 1 pkg. oyster mushrooms, sliced

- ✓ 2 zucchini, sliced

- ✓ 1/2 small yellow onion, cut fine

- ✓ 8 cherry tomatoes, chopped

- ✓ 3 tbs olive oil

- ✓ 1 cup broccoli, cut fine

- ✓ 1 small red and green pepper, chopped.

Procedure:

i. Put essential olive oil in heated stainless wok

ii. add tomatoes and onions

iii. add your chosen seasonings and sauté for 3-4 min

iv. add mushrooms and sauté for another 3-4 min

v. add zucchini, bell peppers, broccoli and sauté 3-4 minutes.

Wild Rice

- ✓ Wild rice
- ✓ Spring water
- ✓ 1 medium yellow onion chopped fine
- ✓ 1 small red pepper
- ✓ 1 cup mushrooms, sliced medium, fine (oyster or brown button)
- ✓ 1/8 cup essential olive oil
- ✓ 1 tsp. thyme
- ✓ 2 tsp. oregano
- ✓ 1 tsp. sea salt
- ✓ 1/8 tsp. African red pepper.

Procedure:

i. Soak rice in spring water till the following

morning for best results.

ii. Cook rice according to package instructions and reserve

iii. pour essential olive oil in hot skillet

iv. Sauté vegetables and mushrooms for 2-3 minutes

v. Add thyme, oregano, sea salt, and African red pepper

vi. Pour in Cooked rice and simmer for 20 minutes.

Tip: *If you forget to soak rice overnight:*

i. Parboil rice for 20 minutes and leave loosely covered until grain opens (approx. 2-3 hours)

ii. Rinse and cook until tender

Or:

Boil grain, adding additional normal water and

stirring as needed until tender.

Spaghetti Recipe

Stick to directions on the Vita Spelt Pasta box about how to cook the pasta.

After cooking the pasta, drain it.

- ✓ In another pan add 1/2 cups of olive oil
- ✓ 2 cups of tomato sauce
- ✓ add 4 tbs of sea salt
- ✓ 1/2 tbs of onion powder
- ✓ 2 tbs of cayenne/chili powder
- ✓ 3 tbs of maple syrup
- ✓ Heat sauce on medium high for ten minutes
- ✓ Stir pasta into sauce
- ✓ Let cook for five minutes.

- ✓ Serve and Enjoy!

Lasagna

- ✓ 1 red bell pepper, chopped
- ✓ 1 yellow onion chopped
- ✓ 2 tbs olive oil
- ✓ Bay leaf, crumbled
- ✓ Spelt lasagna pasta
- ✓ 2 lb., mushrooms
- ✓ 8 fresh tomatoes
- ✓ Almond cheddar cheese
- ✓ Oregano to taste
- ✓ Sea salt, to taste.

Procedure:

Tomato sauce

i. Heat Skillet and add essential olive oil

ii. Place onion, bell peppers, oregano, sea salt, and bay leaf in skillet and sauté

iii. Boil tomatoes for ten minutes

iv. Place in normal ice water for 5 minutes, drain and remove skin from tomatoes

v. Blend tomato in blender -fresh tomato sauce

vi. Add tomato sauce in skillet with sautéed seasonings

vii. Simmer for 30-45 minutes

viii. Set aside half of the sauce to be utilized in the making of the mushroom sauce, remaining half to be utilized when layering.

Mushroom sauce

    i.   Place mushrooms in normal water, soak for 1 minute, strain and slice

    ii.   Season to taste, sauté for 2 minutes and add half of saved sauce (see above), reserve for layering.

Pasta

    i.   Prepare pasta according to instructions

    ii.   Once pasta is performed, place under cool water for easy handling

    iii.   Layer a deep baking dish with tomato sauce

    iv.   Place a layer of pasta on top, then a layer of mushroom sauce

    v.   Then add a layer of almond cheddar

    vi.   Repeat steps until the dish is nearly full

    vii.   Place 2 cups of sauce together with the remainder of almond cheddar

viii. Bake in 350 degree oven for 20 minutes until almond cheddar is melted.

Hot Veggie Wrap

- ✓ 3 cups of diced tomatoes
- ✓ 2 cups of onion
- ✓ 1 cup of diced bell peppers
- ✓ 1/2 cups of mushrooms chopped

Procedure:

i. Stir fry all vegetables for five minutes

ii. Warm spelt tortilla

iii. Put together

iv. Enjoy!

Taquitos

- ✓ 2 cups of chopped onion
- ✓ 4 cups of chopped mushrooms
- ✓ 2 tsp of chili powder
- ✓ 3 tbs of sea salt
- ✓ 2 tbs of tomato sauce
- ✓ 2 tbs of oregano
- ✓ 2 tsp. onion powder
- ✓ 2 tsp. ground thyme

Procedure:

i. Put half cup of olive oil into the pan

ii. Add onion sauté until golden brown

iii. Add mushroom sauté for five minutes

iv. Then add seasonings

v. Wrap in corn shells tightly

vi. Then fry until crispy

Mushroom Salad

- ✓ 1/4 bunch fresh spinach, torn
- ✓ 1/4 bunch red leaf lettuce, torn
- ✓ 1/4 bunch romaine lettuce, torn
- ✓ 1/2 lb. fresh mushrooms
- ✓ 1/2 red bell pepper, chopped
- ✓ 1 sm. red onion, diced
- ✓ 1/2 cup essential olive oil
- ✓ 1/4 cup fresh lime juice

- ✓ 1/2 tsp. dill
- ✓ 1/2 tsp. basil
- ✓ 1/2 tsp. sea salt.

Procedure:

i. Thoroughly wash mushrooms, dry and slice

ii. Add onion, bell pepper, olive oil, lime juice, dill, sea salt and basil

iii. Marinade for half an hour in the refrigerator

iv. Thoroughly wash greens, dry, and shred

v. Add greens with mushrooms and mix thoroughly

vi. Enjoy!

Vegetable Salad

- ✓ 1/2 lb. fresh string beans (Remove ends and snap in two)

- ✓ 1/2 bunch romaine lettuce, torn
- ✓ 1/2 bunch watercress, torn
- ✓ 1/2 bunch cilantro, chopped fine
- ✓ 1/2 tsp. dill
- ✓ 1/4 tsp. cumin
- ✓ 1/4 cup fresh lime juice
- ✓ 1/2 cup olive oil
- ✓ Nice basil to taste.

Procedure:

i. Pour essential olive oil in bowl

ii. Add dill, cumin, basil, and lime juice

iii. Marinade in refrigerator for one and half hours

iv. Mix thoroughly with lettuce, watercress, and cilantro

v. Enjoy!

Avocado Dressing

- ✓ 3 Ripe avocados, peeled and seeded
- ✓ 1/2 small red onions
- ✓ 1/2 tomatoes peeled
- ✓ 1/4 cup fresh lime juice
- ✓ 4 tbs pure essential olive oil
- ✓ Pinch Cayenne Pepper
- ✓ Few sprigs of cilantro
- ✓ 1 tsp. chili powder
- ✓ 1 tsp. oregano
- ✓ 1 tsp. cumin
- ✓ 1/2 tsp. special basil

- ✓ 1/2 tsp. sugary basil
- ✓ 1/2 tsp. thyme
- ✓ 1/4 tsp. sea salt.

Procedure:

i. Puree avocados in blender

ii. Put remaining ingredients and 2 tablespoons of spring water

iii. Lightly blend and pour over your salad.

Note: *Season to taste*

Use cold pressed, virgin olive oil

Creamy Salad Dressing

- ✓ 4 tbs. almond butter
- ✓ 2 green onions
- ✓ 1/4 tsp. ground cumin

- ✓ 1/2 cup fresh lime juice
- ✓ 1/2 tsp. lovely basil
- ✓ 1/4 tsp. thyme
- ✓ 1 tsp. maple syrup
- ✓ 1/4 tsp. sea salt.

Procedure:

i. Inside a glass bottle, add all ingredients and 2 tablespoons of spring water

ii. Shake thoroughly and revel in!

Cucumber Dressing

- ✓ 3 med. cucumbers, peeled
- ✓ 10 almonds, raw, unsalted
- ✓ 4 tbs. Pure olive oil
- ✓ 1/4 cup fresh lime juice

- ✓ 1/4 cup green onions, chopped fine
- ✓ 1/2 tsp. thyme
- ✓ 1/2 tsp. sea salt
- ✓ 1/4 tsp. dill
- ✓ 1-1/2 cup spring water
- ✓ Few sprigs of cilantro, chopped

Putting everything Together:

i. Blend 10 almonds in spring water fastly for 2 minutes,

ii. Strain and set liquid aside

iii. Puree cucumbers in blender with almonds

iv. Add essential olive oil, lime juice and remaining ingredients

v. Lightly blend, adding water, if needed

vi. Pour over your salad and revel in!

Xave's Delight

- ✓ 2 fresh limes squeezed
- ✓ 3 tbs. maple syrup
- ✓ 3 oz. sesame tahini
- ✓ 1 oz spring water
- ✓ 1 tsp. sea salt
- ✓ 1/2 tsp. red pepper

Procedure:

i. Inside a glass bottle, add juice of 2 limes, water, maple syrup, sea salt, red pepper, and sesame tahini

ii. Shake well and dress your salad!!

Lime and Essential Olive Oil Dressing

- ✓ 1/4 fresh lime, squeezed
- ✓ 1/2 cup essential olive oil
- ✓ 1/8 cup spring water
- ✓ 1 tbs. maple syrup
- ✓ 1/4 tsp. special basil
- ✓ 1/4 tsp. thyme
- ✓ 1/4 tsp. oregano
- ✓ 1/4 tsp. ground cumin

Procedure:

i. Put all ingredients in a glass bottle

ii. Shake thoroughly and revel in this scrumptious and easy salad dressing.

Chapter 3

Dr Sebi Food List

Dr. Sebi was a health and fitness guru. A Honduran man with humble beginnings, Dr. Sebi created great strides in the wonderful world of natural health and fitness with the creation of his specialized diet.

Dr. Sebi thought that there have been six fundamental food groups: live, raw, dead, hybrid, genetically altered, and drugs.

His diet essentially cut out all of the food groups except live and raw, encouraging dieters to consume as closely to a raw vegan diet as possible.

This consists of foods like naturally grown vegetables and fruit, as well as wholegrains.

Dr. Sebi thought that the raw and live foods had been

"alkaline," which fought the acidic food waste in your body.

Along with his diet, Dr. Sebi developed a listing of foods that he regarded as the very best for his diet, and named this the Dr. Sebi Alkaline Food List.

Even after his death/demise, the Dr. Sebi product list is growing and evolving.

Sticking with the Dr Sebi Diet and Food List could be difficult in the event that you eat out a whole lot. Consequently, you should get accustomed to preparing a whole lot of meals in the home.

To greatly help with this, we created a Vegan Food for the Soul Cookbook product/gameplan that provides you all the information you have to eat right, plan out meals, and also have fun, flavorful recipes that abide by the diet.

This way there is no need to put an excessive amount of

thought into everything you need to eat and the less thought you need to put into the dietary plan, the easier it'll become to adhere to the diet.

Dr Sebi Food List - Recommended Nutritional Guide

The following is an intensive outline of Dr. Sebi food list.

Dr. Sebi Vegetable List

Much like all his alkaline foods, Dr. Sebi held the belief that individuals should eat non-GMO foods. This consists of fruits and vegetables which have been made seedless, or altered to contain much more minerals and vitamins than they do naturally. The Dr. Sebi set of vegetables is quite large and diverse, with lots of options to produce different dynamic meals. This list includes:

- Amaranth
- Arame
- Avocado
- Bell Pepper
- Chayote
- Cherry and Plum Tomato
- Cucumber
- Dandelion Greens
- Dulse
- Garbanzo Beans
- Hijiki
- Izote flower and leaf
- Kale
- Lettuce except iceberg
- Mushrooms except Shitake
- Nopales
- Nori
- Okra
- Olives
- Onions
- Purslane Verdolaga
- Squash
- Tomatillo

- Turnip Greens
- Wakame
- Watercress
- Wild Arugula
- Zucchini.

Dr. Sebi Fruit List

As the vegetable list is decently lengthy, the fruit list is more restricted, and several types of fruits aren't permitted to be consumed while on the Dr. Sebi diet. However, the fruits list continues to offer fans of the dietary plan a diverse group of options. For instance, all types of berries are allowed on the Dr. Sebi food list except cranberries, which certainly are manmade fruits. The list also contains:

- Apples
- Bananas
- Berries
- Cantaloupe

- Cherries
- Currants
- Dates
- Figs
- Grapes
- Limes
- Mango
- Melons
- Orange
- Papayas

- Peaches
- Pears
- Plums
- Prickly Pear
- Prunes
- Rasins
- Soft Jelly Coconuts
- Soursoups
- Tamarind

Dr Sebi Food List Spices and Seasonings

- Achiote
- Basil
- Bay Leaf

- Cayenne
- Cloves
- Dill

- Habanero
- Onion Powder
- Oregano
- Powdered Granulated Seaweed

- Pure Sea Salt
- Sage
- Savory
- Sweet Basil
- Tarragon
- Thyme

Alkaline Grains

- Amaranth
- Fonio
- Kamut
- Quinoa

- Rye
- Spelt
- Tef
- Wild Rice

Alkaline Sugars and Sweeteners

- Date Sugar from dried dates

- 100% Pure Agave Syrup from cactus

Dr Sebi Herbal Teas

- Burdock
- Chamomile
- Elderberry
- Fennel
- Ginger
- Red Raspberry
- Tila

Dr. Sebi Herb List

The herb list may be the most limited of Dr. Sebi's food lists, since it is difficult to acquire an herb which has not been altered. An excellent guideline for the herbs is usually to think about ones that can be utilized the moment they are picked from the garden (a non-GMO garden, of course). Probably the most versatile herbs on the Dr. Sebi Herb list consist of:

- Basil
- Dill

- Oregano
- Onion powder
- Pure sea salt
- Cayenne

Final Thoughts

Some dieters consider the Dr Sebi food list to be too limiting for his or her liking.

However, faithful supporters of the diet believe that there are enough foods on the list to permit for variety. An average meal with the Dr. Sebi diet might appear something similar to vegetables sauteed in avocado oil on a bed of wild rice, or a big green salad with an essential olive oil dressing. Although it might take some time, the Dr. Sebi's food list could be easy to stick to and good for one's health.

Chapter 4

Dr Sebi Recipes

Dr. Sebi recipes: Its no secret that ingesting healthy can boost your brain and body.

This chapter contains a thorough guide of Dr. Sebi recipes that you can use to maintain a wholesome, alkaline, and vegan diet.

All the recipes below adhere to Dr. Sebi's recommended foods list.

These foods have already been tested and vetted by Dr. Sebi for acidity and alkalinity.

Now lets start with the actual recipes. I've put together the very best Dr. Sebi recipes below to truly get you focused on alkaline healthy living.

Most of the recipes likewise have vegetables/veggies

which can be substituted as meat for a few of your preferred dishes.

My hope is undoubtedly that after studying this chapter, you will make certain that alkaline eating could be fun and exceed eating salads for each meal.

BREAKFAST

Alkaline Blueberry Spelt Pancakes

Ingredients:

- ✓ 2 cups Spelt Flour
- ✓ 1 cup Coconut Milk
- ✓ 1/2 cup Clean Water or Alkaline Water
- ✓ 2 Tbsp. Grapeseed Oil
- ✓ 1/2 cup Agave

- ✓ 1/2 cup Blueberries

- ✓ 1/4 Tsp. Sea Moss

Directions:

1. Mix your spelt flour, hemp seeds, sea moss, agave, and grapeseed oil together in a sizable bowl. (It is necessary you don't introduce the hemp milk now, as it might form lumps once in touch with the grapeseed oil.)

2. Mix in 1 cup of hemp milk and add clean water until you get the consistency you desire.

3. Fold the blueberries into the batter.

4. Heat your skillet to medium heat and lightly coat it with grapeseed oil.

5. Pour the batter into the skillet and let them cook for approximately 3-5 minutes on each side.

6. Enjoy your Blueberry Spelt Pancakes!

If you want the pancakes even more cooked through, you can even try baking it in the oven at 350 °F for some minutes.

Alkaline Blueberry Muffins

Blueberry Muffin Recipe

Ingredients:

- ✓ 1 cup Coconut Milk
- ✓ 3/4 cup Spelt Flour
- ✓ 3/4 Teff Flour
- ✓ 1/2 cup Blueberries
- ✓ 1/3 cup Agave
- ✓ 1/4 cup Sea Moss Gel (optional)

- ✓ 1/2 tsp. Sea Salt

- ✓ Grapeseed Oil

Directions:

1. Pre-heat oven to 365 degrees

2. Grease 6 regular-size muffin cups or line with muffin liners.

3. Mix together coconut milk, flour, agave, sea salt, and sea moss gel in a sizable bowl until blended good, then fold in blueberries.

4. Lightly coat muffin pan with grapeseed oil and pour in muffin batter.

5. Bake for 30 minutes until golden brown.

LUNCH

Chickpea Burger

Ingredients:

This recipe make 3-4 burgers.

- ✓ 1 cup Garbanzo Bean Flour
- ✓ 1/2 cup Onions, diced
- ✓ 1/2 cup Green Peppers, diced
- ✓ 1/2 cup Kale, diced
- ✓ 1 Plum Tomato, diced
- ✓ 2 tsp. Basil
- ✓ 2 tsp. Oregano
- ✓ 2 tsp. Onion Powder
- ✓ 2 tsp. Sea Salt

- ✓ 1 tsp. Dill

- ✓ 1/2 tsp. Ginger Powder

- ✓ 1/2 tsp. Cayenne Powder

- ✓ 1/4 to 1/2 cup Clean Water

- ✓ Grape Seed Oil

Directions:

1. In a sizable bowl, mix together all seasonings and vegetables, then mix in flour.

2. Slowly add drinking water and mix until mixture could be formed right into a patty. Add even more flour if too loose.

3. Pour oil in a skillet and cook patties on medium-high heat for 2-3 minutes on each side. Continue flipping until both sides are brown.

4. Serve on alkaline flatbread and revel in your Alkaline Chickpea Burgers!

Alkaline Flatbread

Ingredients:

This recipe makes 4 - 6 servings.

- ✓ 2 cups Spelt Flour

- ✓ 2 tbsp. Grapeseed Oil

- ✓ 3/4 cup Clean Water

- ✓ 1 tbsp. Sea Salt

- ✓ 2 tsp. Oregano

- ✓ 2 tsp. Basil

- ✓ 2 tsp. Onion Powder

- ✓ 1/4 tsp. Cayenne

The interesting part concerning this recipe is you may

make this in about 20 minutes in fact it is ideal for sandwiches, wraps, or mini pizza.

Directions:

1. Mix together flour and seasonings until well blended.

2. Merge oil and about 1/2 cup of drinking water into the mix. Slowly mix in water until it forms right into a ball.

3. Add flour to workspace and knead dough for approximately five minutes, then divide dough into 6 equal parts.

4. Roll out each ball into about 4-inch circles.

5. Place an un-greased skillet on medium-high heat, flipping every 2-3 minutes until done.

6. Enjoy your Alkaline Flatbread!

DINNER

Vegetable Lo Mein

Ingredients:

- ✓ Spelt Spaghetti Noodles or Kamut Noodles for Gluten free
- ✓ Green Bell Peppers
- ✓ Red Bell Peppers
- ✓ Onions
- ✓ Mushrooms
- ✓ Green Onions
- ✓ Key Limes (optional)
- ✓ Sesame Seeds
- ✓ Toasted Sesame Oil

- ✓ Ginger Powder or Fresh Ginger

- ✓ Sea Salt

- ✓ Grape Seed Oil

- ✓ Agave

- ✓ Onion Powder

- ✓ Red Pepper Flakes

- ✓ Tamarind Concentrate (optional)

Vegan Flatbread Pizza

Ingredients:

- ✓ Spelt Flour

- ✓ Green/Red Bell Pepper

- ✓ Red/White Onions

- ✓ Roma Tomatoes

- ✓ Mushrooms
- ✓ Avocado
- ✓ Oregano
- ✓ Onion Powder
- ✓ Sea Salt
- ✓ Grapeseed Oil
- ✓ Agave Nectar
- ✓ Brazil Nut Cheese
- ✓ Food Processor or Blender.

Alkaline Pizza Crust

Measurements:

- ✓ 1/2 cups Spelt Flour
- ✓ 1 tsp. Onion powder

- ✓ 1 tsp. Oregano
- ✓ 2 tsp. Sesame seeds
- ✓ 1 tsp. Sea Salt
- ✓ 2 tsp. Agave
- ✓ 2 tsp. Grapeseed Oil
- ✓ 1 cup Clean Water

Directions:

1. Preheat the oven to 400°F.

2. Mix all your ingredients together in a medium-sized bowl, adding only 1/2 cup of clean water. Introduce clean water slowly until you can mix the dough right into a ball; Add more flour if an excessive amount of water was used.

3. Lightly coat your baking sheet with grape seed oil,

add flour to the hands, and roll out the dough into the baking sheet.

4. Brush the crust with grape seed oil and poke holes in it with a fork. Bake the crust for 10-15 minutes.

5. Make ready your tomato or avocado pizza sauce as the crust is baking. (Recipes Below)

6. After the crust is ready, add your pizza sauce, Brazil nut cheese*, mushrooms, peppers, and onions. Bake the pizza for 15-20 minutes.

7. Enjoy your Alkaline Veggie Pizza!

NB: *The nut cheese really helps to cook the toppings while baking, if you don't have any nut cheese I would recommend lightly sauteing the toppings before baking.*

Tomato Pizza Sauce

Measurements:

- ✓ 5 Roma Tomatoes

- ✓ 2 tbsp of chopped Onion

- ✓ 1 tsp. Sea Salt

- ✓ 1 tsp. Onion Powder

- ✓ 1 tsp. Oregano

- ✓ 2 tbsp. Agave

- ✓ 2 tbsp. Grape Seed Oil

- ✓ pinch of Basil

Directions:

1. To remove the skin layer, make small x-shaped cuts on the ends of 5 plum tomatoes and place them in boiling water for 1 minute.

2. Put the tomatoes in ice-cold water for 30 seconds therefore the skin could be easily peeled.

3. Blend the tomatoes and other ingredients in your meal processor or blender for 30 seconds or until smooth.

Avocado Pizza Sauce

Measurements:

- ✓ 1 Avocado

- ✓ 2 tbsp. choppedOnion

- ✓ 1/2 tsp. Onion Powder

- ✓ 1/2 tsp. Sea Salt

- ✓ 1/2 tsp. Oregano

- ✓ pinch of Basil

Directions:

1. Slice the avocado down the center, take away the pit, and scrape the insides into your meal processor.

2. Add the others of your ingredients to the meals processor and blend it for three minutes or until smooth, scraping the within of the processor if needed.

Brazil Nut Cheese

Ingredients:

This recipe makes about 6 cups of cheese.

- ✓ 1 lb. soaked Brazil nuts
- ✓ 1/2 of the lime, juiced
- ✓ 2 tsp. sea salt

- ✓ 1 tsp. onion powder
- ✓ 1/2 tsp. cayenne
- ✓ 1/2 cup Hemp Milk, Cashew Milk, or another Nut
- ✓ 1-1/2 cups clean water
- ✓ 2 tsp. grapeseed oil
- ✓ blender or food processor

NB: *It is most beneficial to soak the Brazil nuts overnight, but if you don't have that sort of time, soaking them for approximately 2 hours is merely fine.*

Directions:

1. Add all of your ingredients to your meal processor or blender, excluding the clean water.
2. Adding only 1/2 cup of water, blend the

ingredients together for 2 minutes.

3. Continue steadily to add 1/2 cups of water and blend before desired consistency is reached.

4. Enjoy your Alkaline Brazil Nut Cheese!

Vegan Alkaline Ribs

Ingredients:

This recipe makes 1 serving per mushroom.

- ✓ 2 portobello mushrooms
- ✓ 1/2 cup Alkaline Barbecue Sauce
- ✓ 1/4 cup clean water
- ✓ 1 tsp. sea salt
- ✓ 1 tsp. onion powder
- ✓ 1/2 tsp. cayenne

- ✓ grapeseed oil

- ✓ basting brush

- ✓ cast-iron griddle

- ✓ Skewers (optional)

This recipe may also be made on the grill, cooked in a skillet, or baked at 350°F for 10-15 minutes (after step 4).

If you don't have skewers, you can always cook the mushrooms like riblets

Directions:

1. Scrape gills off the lower of the mushroom cap in order to avoid an earthy taste and slice mushrooms into 1/2 inches apart.

2. Put mushrooms in a sizable container and add seasonings, water, and the majority of the barbecue

sauce.

3. Cover with a lid, shake, and store in refrigerator for approximately 6-8 hours. Flip container over every 2 hours.

4. Take a skewer and add 3 mushrooms to the center, with other skewer, then bring about 2-3 more pieces. If any pieces break, you can cook them as tablets.

5. On medium heat, brush griddle with oil, and cook ribs for 12-15 minutes, flipping every three minutes. Brush with an increase of barbecue sauce if preferred every few flips.

Alkaline Barbeque Sauce

Ingredients:

This recipe makes about 8-10 oz. of barbecue sauce.

- ✓ 6 Plum Tomatoes
- ✓ 2 tbsp. Agave
- ✓ 1/4 cup Date Sugar
- ✓ 1/4 cup White Onions, chopped
- ✓ 2 tsp. Smoked Sea Salt/Sea Salt
- ✓ 2 tsp. Onion Powder
- ✓ 1/2 tsp. Ground Ginger
- ✓ 1/4 tsp. Cayenne Powder
- ✓ 1/8 tsp. Cloves
- ✓ Blender
- ✓ Hand Mixer

Directions:

1. Add all ingredients except date sugar and blend

until smooth.

2. Pour blended ingredients and date sugar right into a saucepan at medium-high heat and stir occasionally until boiling.

3. Reduce heat to a simmer and cover with a lid for a quarter-hour, stirring occasionally.

4. Use stick blender to help make the sauce smoother.

5. Simmer on low heat for ten minutes or until water cooks off.

6. Allow the sauce to cool and thicken further before serving.

7. Enjoy your Alkaline Barbecue Sauce!

The difficult part about been fit with perfect wellness involves knowing things to eat and adhering to the Dr.

Sebi diet program consistently over an extended time frame.

Herbalist and natural healing practitioner Dr. Sebi, committed his life to studying foods and evaluating foods that people take into their body.

Predicated on his life's work, Dr Sebi has come up with a food list to live by and Dr Sebi's recipes are rooted within an African diet that targets alkaline foods that are truly natural rather than acidic.

The recipes can make it easier that you can live a wholesome life and put less thought into the dishes which can be prepared when you aren't in the mood for salad.

The less thought you need to put into everything you can eat, the simpler it'll be for you to remain focused on living healthy.